Dietary Fiber

Your Guide to a Healthy Gut

By PROSENCE

Respective authors own all copyrights not held by the publisher.

The information herein is offered for informational purposes solely, and is universal as so. The presentation of the information is without contract or any type of guarantee assurance.

The trademarks that are used are without any consent, and the publication of the trademark is without permission or backing by the trademark owner. All trademarks and brands within this book are for clarifying purposes only and are the owned by the owners themselves, not affiliated with this document.

ABOUT PROSENCE
Our Mission

We are dedicated to guiding, motivating and providing the tools necessary to transform people into the best version of themselves. Our goal is to empower men and women across the globe to realize that physical and mental fitness are not a short-term solution, but a lifetime choice, and to actualize what they have come to understand into a daily routine. We invite you to discover this process for yourself as you join us in the exploration of science-based knowledge that can lead to better health, greater fulfilment and astonishing vitality.

Who is Prosence?

Prosence is led by Antonio Mazzotta, a strapping 28-year-old Italian health enthusiast who resides in Switzerland. He's a self-described "Mr. Nice Guy" who, (despite a powerful love for his mamma's pasta and pizza), has developed a life dedicated to health and fitness. Now, he strives to share his secrets with the world.

Antonio discovered his passion for health and fitness 7 years ago and has never looked back! Days are filled with working new routines at his gym, training hard, meeting like-minded people and, dear to his heart, teaching weight training, dieting, and healthy lifestyle choices to his valued clients. Job one is helping people to achieve their overall fitness goals, including providing a gain in endurance and a new (sustainable) vitality.

He and his team fight to counter the preponderance of bad information that proliferates the Internet, being driven by offering people a safe yet powerful path to vibrant, brilliant health. In short, *Prosence* is fervently dedicated to the motivation, inspiration and education of people via the dissemination of the real science-based information they need to get into great shape and to stay healthy for a lifetime.

Discover today how we can help you to grow into what you were meant to be and to embrace life to the fullest with newly realized passion!

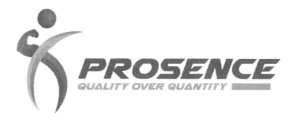

Table of Contents

Introduction

I want to thank you and congratulate you for purchasing the book, *"Dietary Fiber: Your guide to a healthy gut."*

How many of us really pay attention to what we eat? How many of us truly know the different nutrients that our bodies require? If you do, are you all making a conscious effort to meet these requirements?

A balanced diet helps in promoting a healthy lifestyle. I know we all love our fried chicken, bacon and ribs. While it is important for us to appease our taste buds, it is equally important for us to meet our nutrition requirements. This is crucial for the effective functioning of the various organs in the human body.

While most of us focus on carbohydrates, fats and proteins, there is another important nutrient, which we should not be avoiding. That is fiber! If you are not sure what fiber is and which foods contain fiber, don't worry! You have done the right thing by purchasing this book. This book contains all the information you will need to know about dietary fiber, starting from what it means and its types to the various benefits you can enjoy by adding it to your diet. You will also realize how dietary fiber plays an important role in keeping various chronic disorders at bay and helps you lead a healthy lifestyle. There are separate chapters dedicated to help you identify foods which contain fiber and also fiber supplements, in case your lifestyle does not permit you to drastically change your dietary habits.

I am sure that by the end of this book, you will definitely appreciate this nutrient better! I thank you for purchasing this book and I hope you will find it interesting!

Chapter 1
Soluble Vs. Insoluble Fiber

This chapter will give you a brief overview about what fiber is and the different types of fiber. Let's dig in.

Dietary fiber

Dietary fiber is nothing but the portion derived from the plants that we consume, which is indigestible. This is where fiber differs from other nutrients, such as fat, carbohydrates and proteins, which are easily absorbed by the body. Fiber is instead pushed through the digestive tract into the intestines and the colon and finally out of your body.

There are two types of fibers – soluble fiber and insoluble fiber. Let's look at each of these types in detail.

Soluble fiber

As the name suggests, soluble fiber is capable of getting dissolved in water. When this fiber dissolves in water, you get a gel-like product. Foods that are packed with soluble fiber include beans, nuts, apples, blueberries and oatmeal.

Some of the key benefits of consuming foods rich in soluble fiber are as follows:

- Soluble fiber is capable of lowering your blood sugar levels. It is, in fact, capable of improving your body's ability to control glucose, which significantly reduces your risk factors of getting diabetes. There is a separate chapter dedicated to how fibers are capable of affecting your blood sugar levels.

- Soluble fiber is also capable of lowering your cholesterol levels. When dissolved, the soluble fiber attaches itself to the cholesterol particles present in your blood stream. As part of the digestion process, the fiber (along with the cholesterol particles) gets flushed out of the body. This helps in bringing down your cholesterol levels. In fact, oatmeal has proven to improve your overall cardiac health.

- Soluble fiber helps in making you feel full easily. Hence, you won't have to eat too much and worry about putting on more weight. When you feel full easily, you automatically end up eating fewer calories than before. This will most certainly help you lose those extra pounds.

- Because of its nature, soluble fiber absorbs water, as the various organs in your body process it. This helps in adding more weight to your stool and helps you keep both diarrhea and constipation at bay. In fact, most of the fiber supplements available on the market today, contain more soluble fiber than insoluble fiber.

Insoluble fiber

As the name suggests, this fiber does not get dissolved in water. It is more inert in nature and serves as a bulking agent. This type of fiber is mostly found in the peels of fruits and vegetables, brown rice, seeds, wheat bran and whole wheat bread. This is why it is important that you don't throw away the peels of fruits and vegetables.

Some of the key benefits of consuming insoluble fiber are as follows:

- Similar to soluble fiber, insoluble fiber also helps in losing weight. It makes you feel full easily; thereby helping you watch your calories.

- Consumption of insoluble fiber also helps in regulating your bowel movements. If you are suffering from constipation, intake of insoluble fiber can easily help you address that. Several studies have indicated how insoluble fiber plays an important role in effectively handling bowel related disorders, such as hemorrhoids, fecal incontinence and constipation.

Striking a balance

It is important that you consume adequate amounts of both soluble and insoluble fibers. Both these types of fibers are required to improve your gut health and effective functioning of your digestive system. There is a separate chapter which specifies the minimum intake requirement for fibers. This includes both your soluble and insoluble fiber. The several benefits of including fibers as part of your diet, can be enjoyed only if you consume both soluble and insoluble fibers in a consistent manner.

I am sure you now have a fair idea about fibers and the two major types of fibers, along with their benefits. Let's discover in the ensuing chapters the impact fibers have on your overall health.

Chapter 2
Fiber's Role with Digestion

In this chapter, we are going to take a look at the important role that fiber plays in the human digestive process. We will see a broad outline of the digestive system so that you will be able to better understand and appreciate the benefits of including fiber as part of your diet, in the right context.

Digestion process

The process of digestion in human beings takes about 24 hours to a maximum of 72 hours. It happens inside the digestive tract that begins from the mouth and ends in the anus. Now, let us get a little more serious with the science here, shall we? The entire process of digestion can be broken down into three distinct phases; namely the Cephalic phase, the gastric phase and, finally, the intestinal phase. The last two phases, as the names suggest, refer to the digestive process that take place in the gastric region (mouth and stomach) and the intestinal regions respectively. For ease of understanding, the Cephalic phase refers to all those processes triggered by the brain, by when we see, smell or think of food. In this phase, a lot of digestive enzymes and juices are secreted and the body prepares to receive food. As important as it may sound, our area of focus here will be on the gastric and intestinal phases, rather than the Cephalic phase, simply because it is in the mouth, stomach and intestines that fibers work their magic.

Digestion of the food that we place into our mouths starts right there. The teeth and saliva and chewing motion breaks down the large chunks to smaller ones and these are transformed into a manageable (or rather digestible) chunk called bolus, which then travels down the food pipe into the stomach. Inside the stomach, a lot of digestive juices and enzymes act on the food and further break it down for absorption of nutrients, before the food is pushed into the small intestine. It is here, where a major part of the nutrient absorption takes place, aided by the digestive juices secreted by the intestines, pancreas and liver. What is left of the food, which by now is just waste, passes into the large intestine and is stored as feces, before getting passed out of the body.

So, this is basically the digestive process in a nutshell. Having seen that, now let us look at how adding fiber to your diet aids this process. There are certain key areas where dietary fiber aids in digestion and improves the overall health of the digestive tract and, by virtue of that, the entire body.

Role of fibers

You have to understand that the food passes through the digestive tract by means of the bowel movement. These movements happen due to the muscles that line the digestive tract. This operates in a manner very similar to a conveyor belt. By means of constant motion, they move the food from the mouth to the large intestines and out. As you will already know, the body cannot digest fiber and hence it remains as a solid entity in the food inside the body. This increases the mass of the feces, thereby helping it to pass through the gut more easily.

In addition to the benefit mentioned above, the fiber content present in the food also absorbs a lot of water and this slows down the rate of digestion. Because of this, more nutrients are absorbed by the body, especially in the small intestines, which otherwise would not have happened in the absence of requisite fiber.

So, as you can see, including sufficient quantity of fiber in your diet increases the quantity of stool, thereby increasing nutrient absorption and aiding in bowel motion and preventing constipation. When it comes to the large intestine, the benefits of dietary fiber are truly great. Many kinds of fibers are fermented in the large intestine by the bacterial population, which reside in the large intestinal area. The by-product of this fermentation is the production Short Chain Fatty Acids, which have been observed to be beneficial to the colon walls and lining.

In addition to being good for the colon in the manner mentioned earlier, these fatty acids also have a disruptive effect on growth of any undesirable bacterial in the intestines. There are also quite a few research studies that have also shown how these Short Chain Fatty Acids might also be a factor in reducing the incidence of colon cancer. These fatty acids also play an important role in the regulation of blood sugar levels and in the reduction of serum cholesterol levels in the blood.

Furthermore, these beneficial bacteria that live in the intestines, also play a major role in boosting the immune system. In fact, many studies and clinical observations have shown that one of the common symptoms seen in people suffering from acute immune system disorders, is a lack of flora growth in the intestines. These studies can be considered quite accurate since they are based on the study of stool samples of affected patients. Dietary fibers play a significant role in the growth and sustenance of these "good and friendly bacteria." As mentioned above, these bacteria derive the fuel for their existence from the fiber in our diet, hence making the fibers an integral part of their metabolism.

Hence, as you can see, dietary fibers play a major role in digestion in more ways than you may have imagined. They boost digestion, ease bowel motion, increase nutrient absorption and on top of all that, foster the growth of beneficial bacteria in our intestines that quite literally are the reason why our immune systems function the way they do.

Chapter 3
How Does Fiber Affect Blood Sugar Levels?

In this chapter, we are going to see an important benefit of including more fiber in your diet. This chapter will definitely help you understand how fiber impacts your blood sugar levels. Fiber, both in the soluble form and insoluble form, plays a major role in helping you regulate your blood sugar levels and keeping it under control. Needless to say, this is a huge relief for people with any form of Diabetes, who are keen on keeping their sugar levels under check, using natural dietary means. This ability of fiber can also encourage people to include more fiber in their diet, if they want to keep the risk factors of diabetes away. So, let us take a look at the broad ways in which increased quantity of dietary fiber helps to regulate and maintain blood sugar levels and also helps in keeping your body weight under control.

• Reduction in insulin resistance

Many recent studies have shown that consuming food with high fiber content, for a few months, greatly reduces the insulin resistance in the body. There are couple of major reasons that researchers attribute to this aspect of fiber. For one, food sources rich in fiber content have great anti-inflammatory properties. These anti-inflammatory aspects have, in turn, been long associated with reduced synthesis of C-reactive proteins in the blood stream.

The second reason why it helps in addressing your insulin resistance is the fact that fiber in your diet results in production of Short Chain Fatty Acids by the beneficial bacterial flora in the intestines. The secretion of these Short Chain Fatty Acids, in turn, have an inhibiting effect on the body, when it comes to breaking down the fat already present in the body. Now you might wonder what this has to do with insulin resistance. The underlying reason is that a lot of research and studies have observed how the breakdown of the natural fat deposits in the body increases the insulin resistance in the skeletal muscles.

• **Slower release of glucose into blood**

Ingestion of lot of soluble fiber, as part of your meals, greatly reduces the speed with which glucose enters the blood stream, after a meal. There is a strong logic at play here; the higher the amount of soluble fiber in your food, the longer it will take the body to digest and breakdown the food. This means that all that sugar and glucose will slowly enter the blood over a longer period of time rather than hitting you at once! While this definitely holds a lot of benefits in the way you feel after a meal, the overlooked advantage of this is how little stress it puts on the glucose metabolism process. Bear in the mind that this is a great advantage for diabetes patients, whose glucose metabolism processes are already not functioning at the ideal efficiency levels.

• Less glucose produced by liver

As you will see in the next chapter, dietary fibers end up being the fuel source of the healthy bacteria in your gut. The benefits of that process apparently don't just end there. This mechanism aids the body in reducing its glucose resistance. One other beneficial offshoot of this is the reduced production of glucose in the liver. You have to note that the increased glucose production is triggered in the liver, as a direct result of the insulin resistance. So naturally, reduced insulin resistance results in decreased production of glucose!

• Makes you feel full and you eat less

Now this is an aspect that does not need any proof by research or studies! We all know this very well and will have felt how "full" we tend to feel after a meal with good fiber content. It keeps hunger away for long time and you tend to snack less.

There are quite a few simple reasons behind why the body feels this way. For starters, foods which are rich in fiber content, such as cut fruits and green salads with minimal dressing tends to occupy a lot of space in the stomach, even after you have chewed it well. That is because the salivary enzymes and digestive juices in the stomach simply aren't strong enough to break down these fibers. So, you feel full as the stomach is already filled in. This, in turn, makes your brain feel that you have really taken in all the fuel that the body needs.

In addition, as I mentioned earlier, the fiber rich food moves slowly into the gut. This means that all the nutrients in the accompanying food are really well absorbed by the intestinal walls. All this, paired with the fact that fiber rich food generally contains less carbs, means that you feel full sooner, you eat less and, more importantly, you consume a lesser amount of "empty carbs"

• **Tackles obesity**

We all know that obesity is an important risk factor when it comes to diabetes. Maintaining your weight is thus important, if you want to keep diabetes at bay. I have already mentioned how a fiber rich diet helps in making you feel full for a long time. By following a fiber rich diet, you are essentially shutting down your cravings. I think you will agree with me when I say that if we abstain from giving in to our cravings, we definitely can rule out a lot of health issues.

A fiber rich diet helps in tackling obesity in the following manner:

➢ You end up eating less and feeling full for a long period of time. This means that you will be in a position to cut down on your calorie intake, without having to worry about starving yourself.

➢ When fiber accounts for a major chunk of your diet, there is very little room for fat. By reducing your fat intake, you will be able to reduce your weight as well.

➢ We have already seen how fiber helps in dealing with cholesterol levels. Increased levels of bad cholesterol are another contributing factor for obesity. Thus, fiber helps in addressing this root cause for obesity as well.

By addressing obesity, you are thus addressing another risk factor for diabetes!

Chapter 4
Best Dietary Fiber Food Sources

In this chapter, I have compiled a list of 20 foods, which are loaded with fiber. These are easily available and can be incorporated as part of many recipes. Incorporate these foods as part of your lifestyle and reap the maximum benefits.

1. Asian Pears

Asian pears are an excellent source of fiber. They are also loaded with vitamin K, vitamin C, potassium and omega 6 fatty acids. Because of the omega 6 content, Asian pears are instrumental in development of healthy cells and improved nerve and brain function. To get the maximum fiber out of this fruit, eat it with the skin on.

2. Avocados

When it comes to avocados, the fiber content depends on the type of avocado that you're consuming. If you are going for the Florida avocados, which are the bright green and smooth skinned ones, you are in for more insoluble fiber. On the other hand, California avocados, the dimpled and the small and darker ones, do not contain as much insoluble fiber, as the Florida ones. Apart from the fiber content, avocados also pack a lot of healthy fats. This is why avocados are prescribed for lowering cholesterol levels and also for reducing the risk factors for several cardiac diseases.

3. Berries

Both blackberries and raspberries are rich in fiber content. These berries also pack a lot of other vital nutrients. For example, blackberries are packed with vitamin K, which helps in improving your bone density. On the other hand, raspberries are rich in manganese, which helps in promoting the health of your skin and bones and also regulating your blood sugar levels. And the best part is, they are also extremely tasty sources of fiber.

4. Figs

Figs have equal amounts of both soluble and insoluble fiber. Go for fresh figs or dried ones to meet your fiber requirements. In addition to being a rich source of fiber, figs also help in lowering your blood pressure levels and prevent macular degeneration. You can add this fruit to your salad or cereals or even eat them fresh, with some honey or goats cheese. It is one of the easiest sources of fiber that you can really bank on.

5. Coconut

Not many are aware that coconut and coconut products are loaded with more fiber than your oat bran. Coconuts are extremely easy to incorporate as part of your diet. You can either eat them as is, without cooking them, or prepare Asian themed foods, incorporating coconut or coconut products. Another advantage of incorporating coconuts is that they have low glycemic index and they also help in regulating your cholesterol levels. To consciously incorporate coconuts as part of your diet, you can use coconut flour instead of other flours, while baking.

6. Peas

Who would have thought that these innocent looking peas contain so much fiber? Green peas mostly contain a lot of insoluble fiber. Apart from this, they are also loaded with anti-inflammatory agents and powerful antioxidants, which are capable of promoting wellness. You can also get your daily quota of vitamin C, by incorporating peas as part of your diet.

7. Artichokes

Artichoke is a vegetable, which is grossly underappreciated. They are loaded with fiber and are low on calorie content, which make them an attractive addition to your diet. In fact, one medium artichoke is capable of helping you meet almost half your fiber requirements for the day! Hence, if you are not in the mood to assess if you have incorporated several fiber rich foods, you can just keep it simple and incorporate artichokes as part of your meal! Another added advantage of incorporating artichokes, as part of your diet, is that they are loaded with antioxidants.

8. Okra

It is time for you to start looking at okra as a staple food! The benefits of including okra as part of your diet are several, the top ones being its rich fiber content and calcium content. One cup of okra packs so much fiber and three cups of it, every day, is sufficient to meet your fiber requirements for the day! There are so many stew and soup recipes, which hero the okra. You can also look up Asian inspired recipes, which glorify the okra!

9. Brussels sprouts

Oh yes, any list of healthy foods would be incomplete without including the Brussels sprouts. I am sure this is not the first time you have read about the benefits of Brussels sprouts. They are extremely rich in terms of fiber content and are packed with anti-inflammatory agents and antioxidants. Is it time to detoxify your body? Keep it simple and just incorporate Brussels sprouts. There are studies which also indicate that this humble vegetable is capable of preventing certain types of cancer! Do you even need another reason to add this to your shopping cart?

10. Acorn squash

All kinds of squashes (butternut, pumpkin, winter, acorn and spaghetti) are packed with all sorts of nutrients, including fiber. They are loaded with high amounts of soluble fiber. This means, your body has the time to absorb all the nutrients present in your meal. There are some amazing soup recipes out there which can be used to incorporate squashes as part of your diet.

You can also get your hands on a spiralizer and make a salad out of these vegetables!

11.   Turnips

Turnips hardly figure in the American cuisine, which is a sad story! Turnips are packed with so much fiber and contain other nutrients like magnesium, calcium, potassium and vitamin C. You can cook turnips or even eat them raw and get your quota of fiber.

12.   Black beans

Black beans pack a lot of protein and fiber. At the same time, they are also rich in other nutrients, such as manganese, magnesium, phosphorous, thiamin and folate. One cup of these delicious beans can provide you almost 12 grams of fiber! These beans are also loaded with antioxidants and flavonoids, which help in dealing with your risk factors for inflammatory disorders and certain types of cancers.

13.   Lima beans

Lima beans are another easily available source of fiber. Apart from fiber, these beans are also packed with protein, phosphorous, manganese, copper and iron. In fact, a cup of lima beans is capable of helping women meet a quarter of their daily requirement for iron. You also have lots of antioxidants in these beans, which helps in protecting your body against free radicals.

14.   Chickpeas

Who doesn't enjoy a cup of chickpeas? Chickpeas are excellent sources of fiber and the best part is they are extremely delicious and can be used in different recipes. They are also loaded with other nutrients, such as, manganese, protein, omega 6 fatty acids, omega 3 fatty acids and copper. You can incorporate chickpeas as part of your lunch or dinner or even your snacks!

15.   Nuts

Nuts are another excellent source of fiber. In fact, almonds and walnuts pack more fiber than the other nuts. Walnuts and almonds are capable of helping you increase your intake of fiber quickly. Almonds don't contain as many calories as walnuts and also contain lesser fat when compared to walnuts. Another added advantage of including almonds as part of your meals is that, they are rich in proteins and potassium. On the other hand, walnuts are capable of improving your cognitive functions. The best thing about nuts is that you don't even have to cook them. You can just top your cereal or your pasta with some chopped nuts and enjoy!

16.   Lentils

Lentils are fiber rich foods, which are also loaded with folate. A cup of cooked lentils can contribute almost 10 grams of fiber. There are several soup and pilaf recipes available, which are capable of putting the lentils to best use!

17.   Split peas

A cup of cooked split peas is capable of packing around 16 grams of fiber. Split peas are also rich in terms of other nutrients, such as, manganese, protein, folate, omega-3 fatty acids and omega-6 fatty acids. Just a serving of the split peas can easily help you meet around half the recommended daily intake of fiber.

18.   Chia seeds

I know you have already come across the several benefits of this Superfood! They are packed with fiber and help in improving your digestion. Just a tablespoon of these seeds can give you around 5.5 grams of fiber. They can be easily incorporated as part of your diet. Just a word of caution though, while trying to incorporate chia seeds as part of your meals – it might result in bloating or gas for certain people. To prevent these side effects, make sure that you drink lots of water!

19.   Flax seeds

These little seeds are excellent sources of fiber and also contain a horde of other nutrients. They contain proteins, copper, omega-3 fatty acids, magnesium, phosphorous, thiamin and manganese. These seeds are also capable of lowering your cholesterol levels. You can easily add them to your diet as a topping to your salad or as part of your smoothie or as garnish to your soups!

20. Quinoa

Quinoa has proven to be a rich source of fiber. Apart from being a fiber rich food, quinoa is also extremely nutritious. It is easier for your body to digest quinoa, when compared to the other grains. Another added advantage of quinoa is that it is gluten free! Quinoa is also an important source of magnesium, which helps in promoting your overall health and keeping the risk factors for several cardiac disorders at bay.

These are some of the foods which should definitely form part of your diet, if you are trying to meet your recommended intake of fiber. As you can see, these foods are extremely nutritious and can help address other nutrition requirements and promote good health. Hence, be creative and incorporate as many of these exciting ingredients as part of your meals.

Chapter 5

Guidelines for Dietary Fiber Intake

In this chapter, let us look at the latest dietary guidelines and what's the recommended amount of fiber that you should be consuming!

Dietary guidelines (2015-2020)

One of the important reasons behind the increasing trend of chronic disorders is the under consumption of vital nutrients. Studies have proven that while Americans consume nutritious meals and meet their requirements for most nutrients, there are still certain vital nutrients which are under consumed by the population. Dietary fiber is one of the nutrients, which are consumed in very less quantities and many people find it difficult to meet the Adequate Intake Levels or the Estimated Average Requirement. Other key nutrients on this list are magnesium, iron, calcium, vitamins A, C, E and D and potassium. The reason behind this under consumption of all these key nutrients can be attributed to the unhealthy dietary habits.

The latest dietary guidelines help in addressing this pressing matter, to reduce the risks for various chronic disorders and to promote a healthy lifestyle. These guidelines suggest increased consumption of fresh vegetables, fruits, dairy products, whole grains and nuts, which can help in addressing these nutrient deficiencies. As we have already seen in the previous chapter, most of these ingredients are rich sources of fiber. The adequate intake of dietary fiber prescribed by these guidelines is as follows:

- 25 grams of dietary fiber per day – for women

- 38 grams of dietary fiber per day – for men

The below table, as provided in the latest dietary guidelines, helps in identifying the fiber and calorie content of foods, which can be incorporated as part of your diet, to help you meet your dietary fiber intake requirements.

Food	Standard Portion Size	Calories in Standard Portion	Dietary Fiber in Standard Portion (g)	Calories per 100 grams
High fiber bran ready-to-eat cereal	⅓ – ¾ cup	60-81	9.1-14.3	200-260
Navy beans, cooked	½ cup	127	9.6	140
Small white beans, cooked	½ cup	127	9.3	142
Yellow beans, cooked	½ cup	127	9.2	144

Shredded wheat ready-to-eat cereal (various)	1-1 ¼ cup	155-220	5.0-9.0	321-373
Cranberry (roman) beans, cooked	½ cup	120	8.9	136
Adzuki beans, cooked	½ cup	147	8.4	128
French beans, cooked	½ cup	114	8.3	129
Split peas, cooked	½ cup	114	8.1	116

Chickpeas, canned	½ cup	176	8.1	139
Lentils, cooked	½ cup	115	7.8	116
Pinto beans, cooked	½ cup	122	7.7	143
Black turtle beans, cooked	½ cup	120	7.7	130
Mung beans, cooked	½ cup	106	7.7	105
Black beans, cooked	½ cup	114	7.5	132

Artichoke, globe or French, cooked	½ cup	45	7.2	53
Lima beans, cooked	½ cup	108	6.6	115
Great northern beans, canned	½ cup	149	6.4	114
White beans, canned	½ cup	149	6.3	114
Kidney beans, all types, cooked	½ cup	112	5.7	127

Pigeon peas, cooked	½ cup	102	5.6	121
Cowpeas, cooked	½ cup	99	5.6	116
Wheat bran flakes ready-to-eat cereal (various)	¾ cup	90-98	4.9-5.5	310-328
Pear, raw	1 medium	101	5.5	57
Pumpkin seeds, whole, roasted	1 ounce	126	5.2	446

Baked beans, canned, plain	½ cup	119	5.2	94
Soybeans, cooked	½ cup	149	5.2	173
Plain rye wafer crackers	2 wafers	73	5.0	334
Avocado	½ cup	120	5.0	160
Broad beans (fava beans), cooked	½ cup	94	4.6	110
Pink beans, cooked	½ cup	126	4.5	149

Apple, with skin	1 medium	95	4.4	52
Green peas, cooked (fresh, frozen, canned)	½ cup	59-67	3.5-4.4	69-84
Refried beans, canned	½ cup	107	4.4	90
Chia seeds, dried	1 Tbsp	58	4.1	486
Bulgur, cooked	½ cup	76	4.1	83

Mixed vegetables, cooked from frozen	½ cup	59	4.0	65
Raspberries	½ cup	32	4.0	52
Blackberries	½ cup	31	3.8	43
Collards, cooked	½ cup	32	3.8	33
Soybeans, green, cooked	½ cup	127	3.8	141
Prunes, stewed	½ cup	133	3.8	107

Sweet potato, baked in skin	1 medium	103	3.8	90
Figs, dried	¼ cup	93	3.7	249
Pumpkin, canned	½ cup	42	3.6	34
Potato, baked, with skin	1 medium	163	3.6	94
Popcorn, air-popped	3 cups	93	3.5	387
Almonds	1 ounce	164	3.5	579
Pears, dried	¼ cup	118	3.4	262

Whole wheat spaghetti, cooked	½ cup	87	3.2	124
Parsnips, cooked	½ cup	55	3.1	71
Sunflower seed kernels, dry roasted	1 ounce	165	3.1	582
Orange	1 medium	69	3.1	49
Banana	1 medium	105	3.1	89
Guava	1 fruit	37	3.0	68

Oat bran muffin	1 small	178	3.0	270
Pearled barley, cooked	½ cup	97	3.0	123
Winter squash, cooked	½ cup	38	2.9	37
Dates	¼ cup	104	2.9	282
Pistachios, dry roasted	1 ounce	161	2.8	567
Pecans, oil roasted	1 ounce	203	2.7	715

Hazelnuts or filberts	1 ounce	178	2.7	628
Peanuts, oil roasted	1 ounce	170	2.7	599
Whole wheat paratha bread	1 ounce	92	2.7	326
Quinoa, cooked	½ cup	111	2.6	120

Source:

https://health.gov/dietaryguidelines/2015/guidelines/appendix-13/

Chapter 6

Dietary Fiber and the Relationship to Chronic Diseases

Several studies have come to light, which indicate that regular consumption of fiber is capable of dealing with the risk factors associated with several chronic disorders. In this chapter, I have compiled a list of some top chronic disorders and how dietary fiber helps in dealing with them.

Cardiac disorders

Cardiac disorders are the top chronic disorders, which plague majority of the American households. When you shift to a diet which is rich in fiber content, your cholesterol levels will automatically be regulated. We all know that high levels of cholesterol are the main culprits, when it comes to heart related disorders. By adding more fiber to your diet, you are dealing with this risk factor in an effective manner. Some of the fiber rich foods are also capable of improving the functioning of your heart. Incorporating more of whole grains ought to do the trick!

Diabetes

Diabetes is another chronic disorder which affects majority of the American population. We have already seen how fiber helps in managing your sugar levels. When your body is able to regulate your blood sugar levels efficiently, you no longer have to worry about diabetes! A fiber rich diet can definitely help you put your worries to bed!

Colon cancer

I think you will agree with me when I say that colon cancer is the one of the deadliest cancer types! Both men and women face equal chances of developing colon cancer. Studies show that one in 20 women and men end up getting affected by either colon cancer or rectal cancer. Making drastic changes to your lifestyle and diet is required to keep this chronic disorder at bay. As already mentioned, some of the foods which contain fiber in large quantities also contain other nutrients and antioxidants. These foods are capable of preventing certain types of cancers, including colon cancer.

Irritable bowel syndrome

Unfortunately, at least 20% of the American population suffers from irritable bowel syndrome. It is one of the most common diseases/disorders related to the digestive tract. Although there is no known cure for irritable bowel syndrome, you will still be able to ease the symptoms. You can easily tackle your symptoms by making changes to your dietary habits. By meeting the minimal intake requirement for dietary fiber, you will definitely be able to feel relieved of majority of the symptoms associated with this disorder.

Chronic Constipation

Chronic constipation is a disorder, where the person suffers either from infrequent bowel movements or has trouble while passing stools. This disorder could exist for a few weeks or even longer, in certain cases. When you incorporate fiber as part of your diet, it will definitely help in regularizing your bowel movements. Increased intake of fiber adds more weight to your stool. This, in turn, helps in quicker movement of the stools out of the body, through the intestines. Hence, a fiber rich diet can help you keep constipation at bay.

Fecal Incontinence

This is also known as the bowel control disorder. When a person is suffering from this disorder, they find it difficult to control their bowel movements and end up passing stool accidentally. This could be solid as well as liquid stool or mucus. One in every 12 American is prone to this disorder and hence, it is important that necessary precautions are taken. While there is no specific age criterion for this disorder, it is commonly seen among adults. As I already mentioned, including fiber as part of your diet will definitely help in regulating your bowel movements.

When you incorporate the adequate amount of fiber as part of your meals, you will definitely be able to address any constipation or diarrhea issues arising from this disorder. Fiber supplements are also capable of addressing this disorder and help you alleviate the symptoms. Although, I would strongly urge you to consume fiber as part of your meals and not resort to these supplements.

Dumping syndrome

Dumping syndrome is the situation, where the foods that you consume, especially the sugar, move rapidly to your small intestine from the stomach. Some of the common symptoms associated with this disorder are abdominal cramps, diarrhea and nausea. This disorder is often seen in people who have undergone a gastric bypass surgery or other surgeries, which involve removing a part of the stomach. An easy way to address this issue is to have five or six small meals a day, instead of heavy meals. Make sure that you incorporate as much fiber as possible into these small meals. Try eliminating sugar from your diet. This means that you have to say goodbye to candies, sodas, juices and other sugary foods from your diet. Try incorporating as much of whole grains as possible. As we have already seen, whole grains are not only rich in fiber but also help in improving the functioning of your digestive system.

Duodenal ulcer

Ulcers are nothing but open sores, which are frequently observed on the internal lining of the stomach or the esophagus or the upper portion of the small intestine. If these ulcers are found on the upper portion of the small intestine, they are referred to as duodenal ulcers. You can deal with this type of ulcer, by incorporating foods, which are rich in fiber content as well as vitamins. Hence, make sure that you consume fruits, whole grains and vegetables in large quantities.

Hemorrhoids

Hemorrhoids are blood vessels which are inflamed. These are usually found on the lower rectum or your anus. These hemorrhoids can be itchy, cause pain and also bleed sometimes. Hemorrhoids are worsened when you have constipation. The harder your stool is, the more pain you will experience while passing stools. The consistency of the stool can also result in bleeding. Hence, the key to managing this condition is to make sure that your stools are not hard and you don't suffer from constipation. We have already seen how a fiber rich diet can help you keep constipation at bay. When you incorporate fresh vegetables, fruits and whole grains, in large quantities, as part of your diet, the consistency of your stools will be smooth. In the long run, this will ensure that there are no hemorrhoids and even if there are, you will not suffer much from the symptoms.

Diverticular disease

Diverticula are nothing but tiny and bulging pouches, which typically form in the lining of the digestive system. These are frequently formed on the lining of the colon. While these pouches are mostly harmless, there is always the chance of them getting infected or inflamed. Any inflammation or infection results in acute abdominal pain, diarrhea, constipation or nausea. These symptoms can be avoided as well as alleviated by reducing the pressure on the colon. Make sure to include at least 4 to 6 tablespoons of wheat bran as part of your meal, every day. The wheat bran helps in softening the consistency of the waste from your digestion and helps in smooth transition of the waste out of the colon. This significantly helps in reducing the pressure on the colon.

As you can see, the benefits of including fiber, as part of your diet, are multifold. You will be able to address the risk factors associated with various chronic disorders at once, by switching to a high fiber diet. Most of the disorders relating to your digestive system can be easily addressed by consuming fiber.

Chapter 7

How Fiber Helps Protect Against Cancer

I have already touched a bit on how fiber helps in dealing with cancer. There are numerous studies which are being conducted to analyze how fiber protects your body against certain types of cancers. This chapter will throw more light on how fiber plays an important role in protecting your body against cancer!

Colon cancer

We have already seen a bit on how fiber helps in tackling colon cancer. In fact, there are numerous studies which establish this connection between fiber and colon cancer. According to these studies, fiber plays an important role in the effective functioning of the colon. When you consume a fiber rich diet, the time taken for foods to pass through the colon is minimized. At the same time, any carcinogens present in your food or your body is flushed out of the colon by the fiber. In certain cases, the fiber helps in reducing the harmful nature of the various compounds found in our foods. By doing this, fiber attempts to protect your body against the risk factors surrounding colon cancer. Further, when the fiber in your food is broken down by the bacteria present in the lower intestine, a compound called butyrate is released. This compound plays an important role in ensuring that there is no tumor growth in the rectum and the colon.

A study published in 2009 showed that people who adhered to a high fiber and low fat diet had fewer chances of contracting colorectal adenoma. Colorectal adenoma is nothing but a benign tumor, which appears in the colon and the rectum. This lesion is almost always followed by colon cancer. Hence, by reducing the chances of recurrence of these lesions in the colon and rectum, the fiber rich diet effectively helps in minimizing your risk for colon cancer.

Breast cancer

Certain researchers are increasingly focusing on how fiber can reduce your risk factors for breast cancer. Increased consumption of whole grains and wheat bran does the trick. We all know how dietary fat is capable of increasing your risk factors for breast cancer. A high fiber diet leaves very little room for fat. Hence, when you switch over to this low-fat diet, you are invariably addressing your risk factors for breast cancer.

Apart from this, there are also certain studies that indicate the role played by fiber in binding estrogen. When there are high amounts of estrogen in our body, it can increase our risk factors for breast cancer. As part of the natural digestion process, your liver ensures that any excess estrogen is filtered out and sent to the digestive tract. The fiber present in your foods ensures that this excess estrogen is flushed out of the body, along with other carcinogenic waste. Hence, by keeping the estrogen levels in our body under control, the fiber rich diet helps in dealing with breast cancer.

Prostate cancer

Prostate cancer is another common type of cancer, which is a big risk factor for men. There have been studies to understand the connection between fiber and prostate cancer. A recent study conducted on mice indicated that a high fiber diet helped preventing the formation of new blood vessels near the prostate gland. By inhibiting the growth of these blood vessels, fibers are capable of inhibiting the growth of prostate cancer. Similarly, a high fiber diet helps in slowing down the rate at which glucose is metabolized by prostate cancers.

Oral, throat and esophageal cancers

There have been researches which indicate that following a fiber rich and vegetarian diet is capable of lowering your risk factors for oral, esophageal and throat cancers. Whole grains, especially, play an important role in reducing your risk factors for these types of cancers. Whole grains are loaded with other nutrients, such as phenolic compounds, antioxidants and certain flavonoids, which collectively protect your body against the risk factors for these types of cancer.

There are several ongoing researches which try to understand how fiber is capable of dealing with the carcinogenic compounds in our foods and protecting our body against different types of cancers. While some of these researches are not yet conclusive, it doesn't hurt to follow a fiber rich diet, considering how it aims to improve your health in a holistic manner.

Chapter 8

Tips to Incorporate More Fiber!

I am sure that by now, you have a fair idea about the different foods which are rich in fiber content. In this chapter, I have provided some additional tips, which will most certainly help you to fit in more fiber into your diet.

Start with the breakfast

Kickstart your day with fiber. Instead of resorting to your regular cereal, try incorporating bran cereal as part of your breakfast. If you are not entirely comfortable with eliminating your regular cereal, you can mix regular cereal and bran cereal on a 50-50 basis. You can also make a smoothie out of the bran cereal, by grinding about a ¼ cup of it along with some almond milk. Also, you can explore the option of replacing your granola with bran cereal, when you are preparing fruit parfaits or yogurts.

Say no to white bread

You already know how whole grains are loaded with fiber and are extremely nutritious. Hence, wherever possible, incorporate whole grains. When you are choosing your bread, go for the types that are either whole wheat or contain whole-wheat flour or some other whole grain. Do not go for white bread! Make sure to read labels, before buying any groceries. This will ensure that you pick only whole grain ingredients for your meals. Replace white rice with wild rice, brown rice or barley. You can also opt for whole-wheat pasta and bulgur wheat. Refrain from using white flour, when you are baking anything. Try using whole-wheat flour while baking. You can also increase the fiber content by adding either wheat bran or oatmeal to your cookies, cakes or muffins.

Add more toppings

Try adding more fiber to your dish by choosing a proper garnish. For instance, if you are preparing your breakfast, you can add some crushed bran wheat or chopped fresh fruits as toppings for your cereal. Similarly, when you are preparing a smoothie, you can top it up with some flaxseed or powdered oatmeal. You can also use grated vegetables as a garnish, while preparing your meal. Hence, wherever possible, it is important that you try adding a fiber rich food as a garnish to your meal.

Choose your snacks

When trying to go on a high fiber diet, try having 5 to 6 small meals a day, instead of having 3 heavy ones. When you space out your meals that way, you are giving sufficient time for your body to absorb all the nutrients. When you are choosing your snacks for the day, go for fiber rich foods. The easiest option would be to go for some chopped fruits or vegetables. You can also have a handful of assorted nuts. Nuts provide you with some quick energy and can make you feel full easily. You can also opt for a cup of baked chickpeas!

Leave the skin on!

Most of us have the habit of peeling all the fruits and vegetables, before incorporating them in our cooking. The skins also have a lot of fiber and hence it is important that you don't throw them away. While preparing the fruit or vegetable for your meal, see if you can clean and use it, without having to peel the skin. For instance, an apple can be eaten without peeling its outer skin. However, you will have to peel the skins off your turnips, to get the dirt off.

Substitute with vegetables

If you are a meat lover, it's time for you to start focusing on your greens as well. You can include vegetables and legumes as a side to your meal. However, if that is not working out well for you, you can try replacing meat with vegetables and legumes. For instance, go for eggplant Parmigiana instead of the chicken one. Add more lentils and legumes to your curry, instead of meat.

Appease your sweet tooth

As I said before, it is important that you let go of processed sugars and other sugary foods. You will have to skip sodas, candies, sweets etc. Don't drink bottled or packaged juices. Try making your own desserts at home. As I mentioned a while ago, try using whole-wheat flour, wherever possible. Add oatmeal or wheat bran or flaxseed to your cookies or muffins, to add more fiber. You can also satisfy your sweet tooth by treating yourself to a bowl of chopped fresh fruits.

Make sure to read labels

Read the labels of your grocery items, before you buy them. Only when you read the labels, will you know the fiber content each item packs. This exercise will help you pick only those ingredients, which are fiber rich. At the same time, you will be able to eliminate sugary foods from your diet.

Keeping your body hydrated

Fibers can be a little difficult for our bodies to digest in the beginning. As a result, some of us might experience bloating or gas, while including fiber as part of our meals. To avoid any difficulties while digesting fiber, it is important that you keep your body hydrated at all times. Drink lots of water to ease your digestion. While drinking water does not add more fiber to your meal, it will help your body to absorb the nutrients present in your meal in a more effective fashion.

Commit to a new ingredient every week

To keep things interesting and also to include foods which are fiber rich, commit to using a new ingredient every week. There are a whole horde of legumes and grains, which you can experiment with. For instance, try incorporating amaranth, quinoa, bulgur or wild rice as part of your meals. Using all these ingredients in one go might actually bore you. Hence, try adding a different ingredient to your meal every week. For instance, if you made something with chickpeas this week, see if you can swap it with kidney beans next week.

I hope you found these tips useful. Take one step at a time. Don't attempt to make drastic changes to your diet from day one. Your body might not be as receptive as you think. Hence, take it slow. However, the key here is to ensure consistency. This way, you are helping your body to gradually adjust to fiber, introduced in incremental quantities, and process it.

Chapter 9
Fiber Supplements

This chapter will provide you a brief overview about fiber supplements. Of course, before you resort to fiber supplements, I strongly suggest you consult with your physician first.

Types of supplements:

This section deals with different types of fiber supplements, which are available in the market today:

Inulin

Inulin is a type of prebiotic fiber, which is capable of bringing about positive changes to the bacterial population found in your colon. This helps in better absorption of the nutrients present in your foods. You can go for Fiber Choice, which contains inulin. Also, Fiber Choice contains 100% soluble fiber.

Methylcellulose (Citrucel)

This is another soluble fiber, which is made of cellulose. Consumption of this fiber will definitely not result in bloating or gas. This fiber is present in products like Citrucel with

Smartfiber. This is available in powder form and contains 100% soluble fiber.

Psyllium (Metamucil)

This fiber is prepared from the plantago ovata plant's seed husks. This contains almost 70% soluble fiber and the rest is insoluble fiber. Hence, you can reap the benefits of both these fiber types by the intake of psyllium. You can look for the supplement, Metamucil, which contains psyllium. This supplement is capable of addressing symptoms related to hemorrhoids, anal fissures, irritable bowel syndrome and Crohn's disease.

Benefiber

Benefiber contains wheat dextrin, which is nothing but a byproduct of wheat. It does not have any unique taste and dissolves easily in cold as well as hot liquids. You can also use it, while cooking, as it does not contain any thickening agent. Hence, you can easily slip this with your meals and consume it. This contains only soluble fiber and hence is best suited for people trying to manage their diabetes. Another added advantage of this product is that, it is gluten free.

Precautions:

Some precautions while taking fiber supplements are as follows:

- As I said before, please consult with your physician before you consume fiber supplements.

- Certain fiber supplements are capable of causing bloating and gas, until your body gets accustomed to them. Hence, if you already have digestive issues, you need to check with your doctor first.

- Fiber supplements are capable of altering the way your body absorbs certain medications. Hence, if you are already on any medications, it is important that you choose the right supplement, which does not have any adverse impact.

- If you are already suffering from diabetes, you need to check before you consume fiber supplements. As I said before, fiber supplements are capable of lowering your blood sugar levels. Hence, if you are on a prescribed dosage of insulin, you might have to revisit this dosage, in light of the reducing sugar levels.

- Make sure that you drink fluids in large quantities. This will help in digesting these fiber supplements, and you no longer have to worry about bloating or gas.

- Take it slow. Don't try to cram in your entire fiber requirement in the form of supplements. Take these supplements in smaller quantities first. Once your body gets used to them, increase the dosage to meet your daily fiber intake requirements.

Conclusion

This brings us to the end of the book. I know that was a lot of information to process. Remember that fiber should never be a negotiable nutrient – I hope that this is one of your key takeaways from this book. Now that you have a fair idea about the different benefits of fibers, you should make a conscious effort to include it as part of your diet. Start leading a healthy lifestyle, with the inclusion of fibers!

I hope you found this book useful and engaging. I thank you again for purchasing this book!

Finally, if you enjoyed this book then I'd like to ask you for a favor. Will you be kind enough to leave a review for this book on Amazon? It would be greatly appreciated!

Don't forget to follow us on Twitter, Facebook & Instagram to get empowered, educated and inspired to become the best version of yourself in life! You deserve it.

Thank you and good luck!

Printed in Great Britain
by Amazon

35783992R00042